KETO CANDY AND GUMMIES

© Copyright 2020 by Zara Elby All rights reserved.

This document is geared towards providing exact and reliable information in regards to the topic and issue covered. The publication is sold with the idea that the publisher is not required to render accounting, officially permitted, or otherwise, qualified services. If advice is necessary, legal or professional, a practiced individual in the profession should be ordered.

- From a Declaration of Principles which was accepted and approved equally by a Committee of the American Bar Association and a Committee of Publishers and Associations.

In no way is it legal to reproduce, duplicate, or transmit any part of this document in either electronic means or in printed format. Recording of this publication is strictly prohibited and any storage of this document is not allowed unless with written permission from the publisher. All rights reserved.

The information provided herein is stated to be truthful and consistent, in that any liability, in terms of inattention or otherwise, by any usage or abuse of any policies, processes, or directions contained within is the solitary and utter responsibility of the recipient reader. Under no circumstances will any legal responsibility or blame be held against the publisher for any reparation, damages, or monetary loss due to the information herein, either directly or indirectly.

Respective authors own all copyrights not held by the publisher.

The information herein is offered for informational purposes solely, and is universal as so. The presentation of the information is without contract or any type of guarantee assurance.

TABLE OF CONTENTS

Introduction 1

CHAPTER 1 - Getting Started On Keto 2

CHAPTER 2 - Sugar and Ketosis 7

CHAPTER 3 - Keto Candy and Gummy Recipes 11

Conclusion 54

INTRODUCTION

This book contains information about getting started on keto, how sugar affects your macronutrient intake, and ultimately your body. It also includes information on just how to keto-approve your all-time favorite sugary snacks.

This book explores sugar and its effects on ketosis. The difference between normal candies and keto candies, and if there really is such a thing as keto safe candies.

The book will touch briefly on the history of candy and its different types. The book aims to teach you that not all sweet treats are bad with just a little twist on the recipe. The book also includes many recipes of sweets that will keep you and your body in ketosis.

CHAPTER 1
INTRODUCTION TO A KETOGENIC DIET

The keto diet continues to rise in popularity and it's not surprising. It is simple and straightforward. It is surprisingly easy to transition from your current dietary plan to a keto meal plan. All it takes is to know which food you should eat and how to prepare it.

If you are planning to go on a keto diet, you only need to remember three important things: eat low-carb, high-fat food, with low to moderate protein. Your body needs to reach a metabolic state called ketosis to enable it to burn ketones using the process of ketogenesis.

Your Macronutrients

The three major types of chemical compound the human body consumes are fats, carbohydrates, and protein. These three provide the bulk of energy to fuel your body's internal functions and maintain your body tissues and cells.

Other than these three, water should also be consumed in as much as the same quantity because it aids the chemical reactions to the energy produced from food.

Carbohydrates and Sugar

The compound that makes up carbohydrates are sugars. It is classified into four groups:

- Monosaccharides, which require very little effort to break down so they are readily available to burn. Monosaccharides are composed of glucose, fructose, and galactose. Glucose is the main source of energy in this kind of carb, which you can find in foods like pasta, whole grain, legumes, etc. You can find fructose in foods like fruits, select vegetables, soft drinks, and honey. Galactose come from dairy products, dried figs, and legumes.
- Disaccharides, which are broken down mainly through digestion in your small intestines. They are composed of sucrose, lactose, and maltose. Sucrose is your regular table sugar and found in sugarcane, fruits, vegetables, and processed sweetened food like yoghurt, desserts, and ice cream. The chemical make-up of lactose is glucose and galactose and found in products such dairy, and processed foods like bread, baked goods, cereals, snacks, and candies. Maltose consist of glucose and found in barley and malt product like cereals, malted beer, malted candies, and malted milkshakes.
- Polysaccharides consist of starch, glycogen, and cellulose. When three or more monosaccharides join, polysaccharides is formed. Starch is composed of glucose and found in foods like potatoes, tapioca, wheat, oats, rice, yams, cereals, breads, pasta, and other starchy foods. Cellulose is found in plant cell wall and cannot be digested by humans. It is the most important source of fiber for the human body. Glycogen comes

from the glucose found in your bloodstream. The liver forms and stores Glycogen, which aids in maintaining blood sugar level.
- <u>Oligosaccharides</u> are short chains of sugars like fructose, galactose, and maltose. Oligosaccharides are natural in starchy vegetables, fruits, legumes, leeks, garlic, and wheat.

Sugar and Ketosis

The ketosis metabolic state has been used mainly as a means to control the blood sugar levels in the body for diabetics. It was not intended to be a diet plan to lose weight. Weight loss is just an added bonus of using the keto diet.

To stay in ketosis, you need to consume total of 50 grams or less carbohydrates in a day. This means, you need to control the amount of sugar you consume in one day. However, the amount of carbohydrates you need may vary depending on your body and activity levels.

How Safe Are Artificial Sweeteners

The keto diet is all about consuming very little carb-rich foods and substituting them with food that is rich in fiber, fats, and protein. This is easy enough to do by eating vegetables, fruits, fish, seafood, and meat. However, this does not answer how you can consume other foods that you eat like desserts, snacks, and confectionaries with ingredients that are primarily sugar.

Researchers have found alternative ingredients to create keto friendly food. To stay in keto, you can substitute whole grain flour with almond flour or coconut flour. You can substitute sugar with artificial sweeteners like monk fruit, stevia, xylitol, and swerve that comes in granulated, powder, and syrup forms.

Almond and coconut flour are made from natural fibrous food but what about artificial sweeteners. Are they safe? Generally, artificial sweeteners are considered safe because they are tested and regulated by international food and drug authorities to make sure they are safe for human consumption. However, if you have pets be wary as some sweeteners are toxic to them.

The Sugar You Use

Any food with sugar as an ingredient is considered added sugar. This sugar is not the natural glucose that comes from natural food ingredients like fruits, starch, and vegetables. Every gram of added sugar you take has an equivalent gram added to your carbohydrate count.

Added sugar includes agave syrup, fructose, glucose, brown sugar, corn syrup, honey, lactose, maltose, malt, maple, molasses, nectars invert sugar, sucrose, granulated, raw, and honey. These sugars are high in carbohydrates and are often the base ingredients of candies and sweet confectionaries.

Alternatives to added sugar are low carb sugar like advantame, aspartame, monk fruit, saccharin, stevia leaf extract, sucralose, and acesulfame potassium. These alternative sugars are have very little sugar content, which makes it a good substitute for those with diabetes. Low carb sugar has a glycemic index of zero.

Sugar alcohols like isomalt, maltitol, erythritol, xylitol, sorbitol, and mannitol have zero sugar content with almost zero calorie content. Sugar free candies and confectioneries often use either one of these as their base ingredient. The most commonly used for baking and candy making are isomalt, erythritol, and xylitol. Sugar alcohol can affect blood sugar levels despite it being sugar free.

Starting Your Keto Diet

With all that said, you can see just how easy it is to start yourself on a keto diet. It does not stop you from eating anything. You do not have to give up eating even your favorite desserts. The key is choosing the right ingredients and staying within the recommended daily calorie intake.

CHAPTER 2
SUGAR AND KETOSIS

The keto diet is all about limiting your carbohydrate intake. This means limiting the amount of sugar you consume in a day. For most people who enjoy desserts and other sweet concoctions, giving sugar up is challenging. If you love sweets, then you probably also love candies and other sugar based treats. Just how much of these sugary treats should you give up to stay in ketosis?

What are candies?

According to a 2016 study, the highest consumption of candy by a person on average is half pound of candy every week or 35 pounds of candy per year. If a fun-size bar of candy is .33 lbs. and an average fun size has 60 to 100 calories, that would amount to approximately 250 to 500 calories a day. That is a lot of calories considering that the daily maximum added sugar recommended to those not on keto is about 100 calories for women and 150 for men.

Candies are sweet confections that use sugar as its main ingredient. These include any sweet confection like gum, chocolates, sugar candy, gummies, lollipops, any vegetable, nuts, or fruits glazed or coated with sugar, barks, and marshmallows.

What are the types of candies?

You are probably familiar with sugar candies, which you can normally buy in stores but there are several classifications of candies:

- Sugar Candies. These candies have sugar as the main ingredient like marshmallows, taffy, and caramel, soft chewy candies like jellybeans, bubble gum, gummies, and liquorice, hard candies like lollipops, candy canes, and drops, among others.
- Fudge candy, which is made from sugar, butter, and milk
- Nut brittles and barks, which is made from nuts and hard sugar candy
- Chocolates like chocolate candy bars, truffles
- Cotton candy

What are gummies?

Candies are either hard, soft, or gummy. Of all the types of candies, gummies are probably everyone's favorite candy next to chocolate. Gummies are chewable candies made of gelatin, sugar, food color, and flavoring and with gelatin as its main ingredient, you can mold it in various shapes and sizes. Gummies originated in Germany during the 1900s and was first made by a man named Hans Riegel. The most popular gummies are the gummy bears and the gummy worms. They come in many flavors like cherry, apple, lime and other fruity flavors. Other flavors include popular soft drinks flavor like cola and root beer.

Is gelatin healthy?

There is much controversy over the use of gelatin as main ingredient for gummies. Gelatin is produced from extensive boiling of skin, bones, and cartilage of animals. Though it may sound unhealthy, gelatin actually contains amino acids that are good for the body. Gelatin is 99% protein, which is one of the top three macronutrients your body requires.

Are gummies keto friendly?

Gelatin is 99% protein so yes but if you are adding sugar, you need to choose a low-carb or sugar alcohol to keep it keto friendly. If you are vegan, you can substitute it with seaweed gelatin called agar.

What are keto candies?

Keto candies use base ingredients of low carb sugars, sugar alcohols, or other keto friendly ingredients. Keto candies can be either low-carb or sugar free. Keto candies are cooked and prepared like regular candies without the added sugar.

Why regular candies are not keto?

Based on the USDA dietary guidelines, a person should consume less than 10% calorie from added sugar based on the recommended 2000 calorie per day intake. This is equivalent to 50 grams or no more than 12 teaspoons of sugar per day.

The American Heart Association recommends a stricter consumption of 25 grams per day or 6 teaspoons per day for women, and 38 grams or 9 teaspoons per day for men. The

World Health Organization (WHO) has reaffirmed it to 6 teaspoons daily.

The daily carbohydrate consumption of those following keto is 20 grams with a maximum of 50 grams per day. The carbohydrate content of 6 teaspoons table sugar is around 25.2 g. That is more than half of the maximum allowable carb intake. Note that this only allude to added sugar and does not include the sugar from other foods. Just imagine one regular candy can kick you out of ketosis. For this reason, any type of regular candy cannot be keto-approved.

CHAPTER 3
KETO CANDY AND GUMMY RECIPES

MIXED NUTS CHOCO CLUSTERS CANDY

Serves: 25

Nutritional Information (per serving):
Calories: 170 | Calories From Fat: 134 | Total Fat: 19.9 g |
Total Carbohydrates: 5.3 g | Net Carbohydrates: 2.5 g |
Protein: 3.2 g

INGREDIENTS:

- 9 oz dark chocolate chips, sugar-free
- 1/4 cup coconut oil, unrefined
- 2 cups mixed nuts, salted

DIRECTIONS:

1. Prepare a silicone baking mat on a baking tray.
2. On a double boiler, melt chocolate chips. Add coconut oil and stir until well combined.
3. Add the mixed nuts and fold into the chocolate mixture until coated completely.
4. On the baking mat, scoop large spoonful of the chocolate nut mixture. Space them out so they don't stick together.
5. Place in the fridge until it sets and serve.

FRESH BREATH MINTS

Serves: 228

Nutritional Information (per serving):
Calories: 3 | Total Fat: 0 | Total Carbohydrates: 1 g |
Net Carbohydrates: 1 g | Protein: 0

INGREDIENTS:

- 1 cup xylitol
- 4 drops peppermint extract

DIRECTIONS:

1. In a medium saucepan, melt xylitol at 300 degrees F.
2. Once melted, lower temperature to 275 degrees F and add the peppermint oil.
3. Spread on a silicone baking sheet and let dry for 24 hours.
4. Break the hardened mixture into serving sizes or approximately 1 gram.

PEANUT BRITTLE

Serves: 4

Nutritional Information (per serving):
Calories: 316 | Calories From Fat: 261 | Total Fat: 29 g |
Total Carbohydrates: 5 g | Net Carbohydrates: 2 g | Protein: 10 g

INGREDIENTS:

- 1 cup peanuts, salted and roasted
- 2 oz butter
- 3 oz swerve sweetener
- 1 tsp vanilla extract

DIRECTIONS:

1. Line a cookie sheet with wax paper and spread out the peanuts.
2. Using a small saucepan over medium heat, combine the butter, sweetener, and vanilla.
3. Cook until it reaches the caramelized stage and is deep brown in color. Do not undercook to avoid making your brittle grainy.
4. Pour the caramel over the spread peanuts and let it cool for 30 minutes to an hour. Once it hardens, break into pieces before serving.

CRYSTAL CANDY SKEWERS

Serves: 10

Nutritional Information (per serving):
Calories: 34 | Total Fat: 0 | Total Carbohydrates: 8 g |
Net Carbohydrates: 8 g | Protein: 0

INGREDIENTS:

- 2 cups water
- 4 cups granulated sweetener
- 1/2 tsp peppermint extract
- 2 drops green food coloring

DIRECTIONS:

1. Wet 10 skewers with water then roll it them in the granulated sugar. Set aside to dry.
2. In a medium size pan, pour the water and bring it to a boil. Add the granulated sweetener one cup at a time while stirring continuously.
3. Boil until the sweetener dissolves.
4. Remove from heat. Add the peppermint and the green food coloring and stir to get an even color.
5. Allow the syrup to cool down for 10 minutes before pouring into the slim glasses.
6. Dip one skewer per glass, using two clothespin to hold your glass straight and steady. Make sure each skewer hangs an inch from the bottom.
7. Place the glasses in a cool place away from sunlight and cover the top loosely with plastic wrap.
8. After two to four hours, crystals will start to form inside the glass. Allow the crystal to grow until it reaches your

desired size. The crystals will expand inside the glass so make sure it does not over grow inside your glass.
9. Crack the crystal gently and pull out the skewer to dry before serving.

PECAN BRITTLE SQUARES

Serves: 24

Nutritional Information (per serving):
Calories: 63 | Calories From Fat: 48.6 | Total Fat: 5.4 g |
Total Carbohydrates: 10.3 g | Net Carbohydrates: 0.9 g |
Protein: 0.2 g

INGREDIENTS:

- 12 pieces choc zero chocolate
- 1/2 cup choc zero syrup, caramel
- 1/4 cup unsalted butter
- 4 tbsp monk fruit, powdered
- 2 oz chopped pecans

DIRECTIONS:

1. Use half of the pecans to fill each square of your brownie square silicone mold.
2. In a saucepan, melt the butter on low heat. One butter is melted, turn the heat to medium-low heat and add the syrup and monk fruit, whisking frequently.
3. Get it to boiling point and wait for the mixture to froth without forming bubbles. Whisk for 30 seconds then remove from heat before whisking for another 20 seconds.
4. Pour over the silicone mold, filling it halfway.
5. Melt the chocolate on a double boiler.
6. Stir in the chocolate and let it cool for a minute or two before pouring over the silicone mold, covering the caramel.
7. Top the chocolate with the remaining pecans.
8. Let it cool to room temperature before wrapping.
9. Serve as a snack or as dessert.

BRITTLE BUTTERSCOTCH CANDY

Serves: 16

Nutritional Information (per serving):
Calories: 102 | Calories From Fat: 108 | Total Fat: 12 g |
Total Carbohydrates: 0 | Net Carbohydrates: 0 | Protein: 0

INGREDIENTS:

- 1 cup butter, grass-fed
- 1/2 cup monk fruit sweetener
- 1 tsp vanilla extract
- 1 tsp pink Himalayan salt

DIRECTIONS:

1. Using a heavy bottom pan, melt butter over medium heat.
2. Add the sweetener and stir often. Bring to a boil and continue to stir.
3. When the mixture reaches boiling point, reduce heat to low.
4. Continue stirring until the mixture turns amber in color.
5. Remove from the heat and stir in salt and vanilla.
6. Cool for three minutes while stirring.
7. Pour in an 8x8-inch pan and put in the fridge at least 8 hours or overnight.
8. Break into pieces before serving.

PECAN CANDIES

Serves: 24

Nutritional Information (per serving):
Calories: 242 | Calories From Fat: 215 | Total Fat: 23.9 g |
Total Carbohydrates: 6.6 g | Net Carbohydrates: 3 g | Protein: 2.4 g

INGREDIENTS:

- 6 tbsp swerve brown
- 3 tbsp allulose
- 5 tbsp butter
- 1/2 cup heavy cream
- 1/4 tsp xanthan gum
- 1/4 tsp sea salt
- 2 cups pecans, cut in halves
- 4 oz dark chocolate, sugar free, chopped

DIRECTIONS:

1. Combine 4 tbsp of butter and the sweeteners on medium heat in a large saucepan.
2. Cook for 3 to 5 minutes or until boiling. Take off of the heat and add the cream. This will make the mixture bubble.
3. Return the mixture to medium heat and wait for boiling point. Boil 3 minutes. Sprinkle the xanthan gum and salt, then whisk.
4. Let cool for an hour. Make sure it is creamy thick and not solid.
5. Preheat the oven at 360 degrees F. Line a cookie tray with wax paper. Spread the out the pecans and toast for 7-10 minutes. After toasting, arrange the pecans in clusters of 3 to 4 pieces.
6. Drizzle each cluster with 2-3 teaspoons of caramel. Make sure there is enough caramel to clump the pecans

together. Place the cookie tray in the freezer and let the caramel harden.
7. In a double boiler, combine a tbsp of butter and dark chocolate. Stir until melted and smooth. Top over the chilled pecans.
8. Sprinkle with salt and let set before serving.

BOURBON CANDY BALLS

Serves: 20

Nutritional Information (per serving):
Calories: 123 | Calories From Fat: 99 | Total Fat: 11 g |
Total Carbohydrates: 3 g | Net Carbohydrates: 1 g | Protein: 1 g

INGREDIENTS:

- 1/2 cup pecans, chopped
- 1/4 cup bourbon
- 1 cup swerve confectioners
- 8 tbsp butter, unsalted and softened
- 2 oz cream cheese, softened
- 2 1/2 tbsp coconut flour
- 3/4 cup dark chocolate, sugar-free
- 2 tsp coconut oil
- 20 pecans, halved

DIRECTIONS:

1. Pre-soak 1/2 cup chopped pecans in bourbon for 24 hours.
2. In a mixing bowl, mix with an electric mixer the swerve, butter, and cream cheese until it turns creamy and fluffy.
3. Add the pecan and bourbon mixture and coconut flour and mix until it becomes smooth. Refrigerate for 10 minutes.
4. After chilling, scoop a tbsp of the mixture on a lined baking sheet and shape it into a ball. Freeze the balls in the freezer.
5. While waiting, prepare a double boiler over medium heat and melt the dark chocolate and coconut oil. Stir constantly until completely melted.
6. Remove the bourbon balls in the freezer and dip them one at a time into the melted chocolate. Then place it back on the lined baking sheet and top with one half of the pecan.
7. Return to the freezer and let it set before serving.

MIXED NUTS CHOCO CANDY CLUSTERS

Serves: 25

Nutritional Information (per serving):
Calories: 170 | Calories From Fat: 134 | Total Fat: 19.9 g |
Total Carbohydrates: 5.3 g | Net Carbohydrates: 2.5 g |
Protein: 3.2 g

INGREDIENTS:

- 9 oz dark chocolate chips, sugar-free
- 1/4 cup coconut oil, unrefined
- 2 cups mixed nuts, salted

DIRECTIONS:

1. Prepare a silicone-baking mat on a baking tray.
2. On a double boiler, melt chocolate chips. Add coconut oil and stir until well combined. Add the mixed nuts and fold into the chocolate mixture until coated completely.
3. On the baking mat, scoop large spoonful of the chocolate nut mixture. Space them out so they don't stick together.
4. Place in the fridge until it sets and serve.

SOFT MALLOWS

Serves: 10

Nutritional Information (per serving):
Calories: 14 | Total Fat: 0 | Total Carbohydrates: 0.1 g |
Net Carbohydrates: 0.1 g | Protein: 1.5 g

INGREDIENTS:

- 1 cup water, divide in half
- 2 1/2 tbsp unflavored gelatin, grass-fed
- 2/3 cup swerve sweetener
- 2/3 cup allulose
- 1/8 tsp cream of tartar
- Pinch of salt
- 1/8 tsp peppermint extract
- Cooking spray

DIRECTIONS:

1. Prepare an 8x8-inch pan and line with wax paper. Spray with cooking spray and set aside.
2. In a mixing bowl, pour half of the water and gelatin. Place the mixing bowl in a stand mixer and let it stand.
3. Prepare a medium saucepan and place it on medium heat. Combine the remaining half of the water, the two sweeteners, cream of tartar, and salt. Stir until the sweeteners dissolve.
4. Bring to a boil at 237 degrees F. Use thermometer to test temperature. Remove the mixture from heat.
5. Turn on the stand mixer on low speed and pour the boiled mixture slowly over the softened gelatin. Add the peppermint.
6. Turn the mixer on medium high speed and mix for 5 to 15 minutes or until the mixture turns lukewarm, thick and white.

7. Immediately pour the mixture on the prepared pan. You have to be fast because the mixture can set quickly. Smooth the top and leave it to set up to 6 hours or until it is no longer sticky to the touch.
8. Flip on a cutting board and cut into desires size. Dust with powder sweetener if desired or simply expose to air until dry.

FLUFFY MARSHMALLOWS

Serves: 8

Nutritional Information (per serving):
Calories: 7 | Calories From Fat: 0 | Total Fat: 0 |
Total Carbohydrates: 0 | Net Carbohydrates: 0 | Protein: 2 g

INGREDIENTS:

- 1/2 cup cold water
- 2.5 tbsp gelatin powder
- 1/4 cup erythritol
- A dash of stevia
- 1/2 cup warm water
- 1 tsp vanilla extract
- A dash of salt
- Coconut oil, for greasing

DIRECTIONS:

1. Prepare an 8x8-inch pan and line with parchment paper.
2. Grease the parchment paper with coconut oil.
3. In a small bowl, combine the cold water and gelatin powder and let it stand for 10 minutes.
4. In a small saucepan, combine warm water, erythritol, dash of stevia, vanilla, and salt. Stir and just before boiling point remove from stove.
5. With an electric mixer, whisk the gelatin mixture and slowly add in the hot liquid.
6. Keep whisking at high speed for 10 minutes or until the gelatin turns white and foamy.
7. Continue to whisk for another 10 minutes until the gelatin doubles in volume. Pour quickly in the pan and smoothen the top with a greased spatula.
8. Put in the fridge overnight.
9. Grease a knife and cut the mallows into cubes before serving.

STRAWBERRY CREAM FUDGE

Serves: 9

Nutritional Information (per serving):
Calories: 93 | Calories From Fat: 72 | Total Fat: 8 g |
Total Carbohydrates: 3.2 g | Net Carbohydrates: 1.3 g | Protein: 1 g

INGREDIENTS:

- 1/2 cup coconut butter
- 1/4 cup milk, non-dairy
- 15-20 drops monk fruit syrup
- 1 tsp vanilla extract
- 3 fresh strawberries, sliced into three

DIRECTIONS:

1. Prepare a loaf pan and line with parchment paper.
2. In a saucepan, melt the coconut butter while stirring constantly. Pour the melted coconut butter into a glass-measuring cup. Add in monk fruit, milk and vanilla. Stir.
3. Transfer the mixture in a loaf pan and smoothen with a spatula. Cover the pan with the sliced strawberry and press gently.
4. Chill for 30 minutes or until firm.
5. Slice into pieces before serving.

CHOCO ALMOND FUDGE

Serves: 60

Nutritional Information (per serving):
Calories: 12 | Calories From Fat: 9 | Total Fat: 1 g |
Total Carbohydrates: 1 g | Net Carbohydrates: 1 g | Protein: 0

INGREDIENTS:

- 2 cups sweetener, granulated
- 1/2 cup cocoa, unsweetened
- 1 cup almond milk
- 4 tbsp butter, unsalted
- 1 tbsp vanilla extract

DIRECTIONS:

1. Spray an 8x8-inch pan with cooking spray then line with parchment paper.
2. In a saucepan, combine sweetener, cocoa, and almond milk. Bring it to a boil.
3. Stir constantly then lower heat to simmer. Once simmering do not stir.
4. Let it simmer to 238 degrees F.
5. Remove from heat then add butter and vanilla. Stir until it does not look glossy anymore.
6. Pour into the prepared pan, let it cool, and set.
7. Cut into 1-inch size before serving.

DARK CREAM FUDGE

Serves: 16

Nutritional Information (per serving):
Calories: 259 | Calories From Fat: 234 | Total Fat: 26 g |
Total Carbohydrates: 5 g | Net Carbohydrates: 3 g | Protein: 4 g

INGREDIENTS:

- 1 cup butter
- 1 oz dark baking chocolate, unsweetened
- 1 cup almond butter, unsweetened
- 8 oz cream cheese
- 1 cup swerve confectioners
- 1 tsp stevia concentrated powder
- 1/3 cup cocoa powder, unsweetened
- 1 tsp vanilla extract

DIRECTIONS:

1. Prepare an 8x8-inch pan and line it with wax paper.
2. In a saucepan over medium heat, melt butter and baking chocolate.
3. Using an electric mixer, blend the almond butter and cream cheese.
4. Remove from heat and stir in the sweeteners and cocoa powder.
5. Combine all mixes in the blender. Blend again using the electric mixer. Add the vanilla while continuing to blend until it is smooth.
6. Spread the mixture on the pan and chill in the fridge until it hardens.
7. Cut into squares before serving.

TOOTSIE ROLL CANDY

Serves: 36

Nutritional Information (per serving):
Calories: 15 | Calories From Fat: 8 | Total Fat: 0.9 g |
Total Carbohydrates: 3.3 g | Net Carbohydrates: 0.4 g |
Protein: 0.6 g

INGREDIENTS:

- 1/4 cup cocoa
- 1/4 cup whey protein, unflavored
- 2 tbsp whole milk powder
- 1/2 cup erythritol
- 1/8 tsp salt
- 3 tbsp Sukrin fiber syrup
- 2 tbsp butter, melted
- 1/2 tsp vanilla extract

DIRECTIONS:

1. Combine whey protein, cocoa, powdered milk, erythritol, and salt in a bowl and mix. Set aside.
2. Heat sukrin fiber syrup in a microwave oven for 30 seconds. Add the vanilla extract and melted butter.
3. Add in the cocoa mix and combine well until crumbly. Knead until it turns into a soft dough.
4. Flatten the dough and cut into strips. Roll the strips into a rope about the diameter of the tootsie roll. Cut the rope strips into tootsie roll sizes.
5. Wrap each roll individually on a small wax paper.
6. Refrigerate until ready to serve.

CARAMEL CHEWY CANDY

Serves: 12

Nutritional Information (per serving):
Calories: 13 | Calories From Fat: 9 | Total Fat: 1 g |
Total Carbohydrates: 3.2 g | Net Carbohydrates: 0.2 g | Protein: 0

INGREDIENTS:

- 2 tbsp choc zero syrup
- 2 tsp monk fruit sweetener, powder
- 1 tbsp butter, unsalted

DIRECTIONS:

1. In a saucepan on low heat, melt the butter.
2. After melting the butter, turn to medium-low heat add the syrup and the monk fruit. Bring to a boil. Whisk often past the boiling point.
3. Once the mixture starts to froth, turn off the heat and continue to whisk for another 20 seconds.
4. Pour in silicone molds and let it cool.
5. Serve as is or wrapped in wax paper.

HARD NOUGAT CANDY

Serves: 12

Nutritional Information (per serving):
Calories: 70 | Calories From Fat: 60 | Total Fat: 6 g |
Total Carbohydrates: 19 g | Net Carbohydrates: 18 g | Protein: 3 g

INGREDIENTS:

- 1 cup macadamia nuts
- 1 cup erythritol
- 2 tbsp water
- 1 egg white, large
- A pinch of salt

DIRECTIONS:

1. Preheat your oven to 200 degrees F.
2. Prepare an 8x6-inch pan and line with parchment paper.
3. In a skillet over medium heat, toast the macadamia nuts until golden.
4. Remove from heat.
5. In a small saucepan, combine water and erythritol. Stir on a medium heat until translucent and simmering, about 20 minutes.
6. While waiting to simmer, beat the egg white and salt until it starts to form soft peaks.
7. Pour the syrup in slowly while you continually whisk the egg whites until they are well combined.
8. Transfer the mix back to the saucepan and keep stirring over low heat for about 30 minutes. Pour over the macadamia nuts.
9. Place the bake pan in the oven for 2 hours to dry the candy.
10. Remove from the oven and allow to cool at room temperature before unmolding and slicing into pieces.

CHEWY SALTWATER TAFFY

Serves: 100

Nutritional Information (per serving):
Calories: 15 | Total Fat: 0 | Total Carbohydrates: 3 g |
Net Carbohydrates: 3 g | Protein: 0

INGREDIENTS:

- 1/2 cup water
- 1 cup light corn syrup
- 2 cups sweetener, granulated
- 3/4 tsp salt
- 2 tbsp butter
- 1 tsp vanilla extract
- 1/4 cup marshmallow cream
- 3-4 drops food coloring

DIRECTIONS:

1. Spray a baking sheet with non-stick cooking spray.
2. In a saucepan over medium-high heat, combine water, corn syrup, sweetener, and salt. Stir until sugar dissolves.
3. With a pastry brush, wash down the side of the saucepan to prevent crystallization.
4. Bring to a boil without stirring until it reaches 255 degrees F to get a soft chewy taffy. Increase temperature by 5 to 10 degrees to get a firm to very firm taffy.
5. Once you reach the desired temperature, remove from heat. Add the butter and vanilla and stir until butter completely melts.
6. Pour the mixture on the prepared baking sheet and spread out.
7. Pour the marshmallow cream and the food color on top.
8. Let the candy cool for 5 to 10 minutes.
9. Fold all edges to the center of the marshmallow cream.

10. Wear food-safe plastic gloves to protect your hands from heat and spray your hands with non-stick spray.
11. Knead the candy until marshmallow cream and food color mix in. Stretch the candy into a rope then bring it back together. Twist the candy and repeat the pulling process.
12. Continue to pull and twist for 20 minutes until it holds its shape well or until you see parallel ridges on the candy.
13. Divide the taffy into manageable working sizes. Roll them into long thin ropes of 1/2-inch diameter then cut them into 1-inch size piece.
14. Wrap in wax paper to keep it from sticking together and serve.

CLASSIC GUMMY BEARS

Serves: 2

Nutritional Information (per serving):
Calories: 20 | Calories From Fat: 0 | Total Fat: 0 |
Total Carbohydrates: 0.01 g | Net Carbohydrates: 0 | Protein: 3 g

INGREDIENTS:

- 0.3 oz packet Jell-O, sugar free
- 0.25 oz packet unflavored gelatin powder
- 1/4 cup water

DIRECTIONS:

1. Prepare gummy bear molds that has 50 molds per tray.
2. Combine all ingredients in a cooking pan. Cook over low heat until powder completely dissolves.
3. Remove from stove the use a dropper to fill up the mold.
4. Once all empty molds are filled, place in the refrigerator around 30 minutes until the gelatin sets.
5. Pop the bears off the tray and serve.
6. You can use different flavor packs of Jell-O and add the same amount of unflavored gelatin and water, then repeat the process.

RASPBERRY SOUR GUMMY BEARS

Serves: 6

Nutritional Information (per serving):
Calories: 19 | Calories From Fat: 0 | Total Fat: 0 |
Total Carbohydrates: 2.2 g | Net Carbohydrates: 1.5 g |
Protein: 2.3 g

INGREDIENTS:

- 1/2 cup water
- 2 tbsp raspberry powder
- 2-4 tbsp allulose
- 1/2 tsp vitamin c powder
- 2 1/2 tbsp unflavored gelatin

For the sour coating:

- 2 tsp allulose
- 1/2 tsp raspberry powder
- 1/4 tsp vitamin c powder

DIRECTIONS:

1. Over medium heat, use a saucepan to combine water, raspberry powder, allulose, and vitamin c and stir.
2. Turn the heat to low and add in gelatin. Stir for 3 minutes or until the powder dissolves.
3. Remove from heat and pour into a bowl.
4. Use a dropper to fill in the gummy bear silicone mold.
5. Allow to cool for 15 minutes before placing in the refrigerator for 30 minutes.
6. Mix all the sour coating ingredients.
7. Coat gummies before serving.

VERY BERRY GUMMIES

Serves: 15

Nutritional Information (per serving):
Calories: 17.5 | Calories From Fat: 0.9 | Total Fat: 0.1 g |
Total Carbohydrates: 1.8 g | Net Carbohydrates: 1 g | Protein: 2.5 g

INGREDIENTS:

- 115 g fresh strawberries, halved
- 80 g fresh raspberries
- 70 g fresh blackberries
- 6 tbsp gelatin powder, grass-fed
- 180 ml cold water

DIRECTIONS:

1. Combine the gelatin and water in a bowl and allow to set.
2. Using a high speed blender, combine the berries and blend until smooth
3. Strain the berries using a muslin cloth. Discard the pulp.
4. Using a saucepan on low heat, pour half of the juice. Add the gelatin and stir until it dissolves.
5. Remove the mixture from heat and add remaining juice. Remove any foam using a spoon.
6. Fill in your gummy bear silicone mold using a dropper or pipette.
7. Refrigerate for 2 hours to set before serving.

ORANGE-STRAWBERRY FRUIT TEA GUMMY SNAKE

Serves: 4

Nutritional Information (per serving):
Calories: 18 | Calories From Fat: 9 | Total Fat: 1 g |
Total Carbohydrates: 0.1 g | Net Carbohydrates: 0.1 g | Protein: 4 g

INGREDIENTS:

- 3 fruit tea bags, orange flavor
- 3 fruit tea bags, strawberry flavor
- 500 ml boiling hot water
- 6 tbsp unflavored gelatin powder
- 4 tbsp stevia

DIRECTIONS:

1. Divide the water, gelatin powder, and stevia in half.
2. Pour 250 ml hot water each in 2 mugs and dip each flavor of tea bags in each mug. Leave to brew until you get a strong flavor or around 2 minutes. Do not let the water cool down.
3. Remove the tea bags while the tea is still hot, add the 3 tbsp gelatin powder and 2 tbsp sweetener in each mug and stir until dissolved.
4. Using a snake silicone mold, use two droppers for each flavor and squeeze the droppers from both ends of your snake silicone mold. This will give you a two-flavor snake gummy. You can fill two snake silicone molds with this recipe.
5. Refrigerate for 1 hour or until gummy sets before serving.

FLAVORED GUMMY CANDIES

Serves: 20

Nutritional Information (per serving):
Calories: 42 | Calories From Fat: 0 | Total Fat: 0 |
Total Carbohydrates: 0 | Net Carbohydrates: 0 | Protein: 11 g

INGREDIENTS:

- 1 package Jell-O lime flavored gelatin, sugar free
- 1.5 oz unflavored gelatin powder
- 1/2 cup cold water
- Non-stick cooking spray

DIRECTIONS:

1. Prepare a candy mold tray by spraying with a light non-stick cooking spray.
2. In a small saucepan, combine the all ingredients and whisk together until well combined and the gelatin powder dissolves.
3. Place the saucepan on stove over medium heat while whisking continuously for 5 minutes.
4. Remove from pan and transfer to a cup with spout.
5. Pour the mixture in each cavity of the candy mold tray and let cool for 20 minutes before refrigerating until fully set.
6. Remove the candies from the mold and serve or store in airtight containers.

MINT GUMDROPS

Serves: 7

Nutritional Information (per serving):
Calories: 30 | Calories From Fat: 0 | Total Fat: 0 |
Total Carbohydrates: 1 g | Net Carbohydrates: 0 | Protein: 5 g

INGREDIENTS:

- 5 cups filtered water
- 2 tbsp dried peppermint leaves
- 1/4 tsp citric acid
- 1 tbsp grated lemon zest
- 6 micro-scoops stevia extract
- 1 pinch turmeric
- 6 tbsp beef gelatin, grass fed
- 1/2 cup water
- 4 drops natural peppermint flavor with E140 color

DIRECTIONS:

1. Infuse the peppermint leaves in 5 cups of water by boiling it for 5 minutes. Cool before straining and transferring to another pan.
2. Place the strained peppermint water back on the stove to heat again.
3. Combine water and gelatin and add to the peppermint water. Stir and let it boil until the gelatin dissolves. Remove from heat.
4. Add the sweetener, citric acid, lemon zest, and turmeric. Mix well until it turns into a golden hue.
5. Divide the mixture into 2. Add peppermint flavor and green food color to the 1 half.
6. Pour the mixture in layers into the silicone mold and put

in the fridge for minimum of 2 hours. The longer it is in the fridge, the firmer your gummy will get.
7. Remove the gumdrops from your mold before serving.

COKE FLAVORED GUMMY

Serves: 5

Nutritional Information (per serving):
Calories: 14 | Calories From Fat: 0 | Total Fat: 0 |
Total Carbohydrates: 0 | Net Carbohydrates: 0 | Protein: 3.5 g

INGREDIENTS:

- 25 g gelatin powder, unflavored
- 1/3 cup boiling water
- 1/2 cup cold water
- 12 drops stevia cola flavor
- 9 drops natural purple food coloring
- 3 drops natural yellow food coloring

DIRECTIONS:

1. In a microwaveable container, place boiling water and add gelatin powder. Whisk then place in microwave for 30 seconds.
2. Remove from microwave and whisk again. Add the cold water and continue whisking to combine.
3. Add the cola drops and whisk. Taste if you wish to add more flavoring. Add both the food colors to get a dark brown color. Place in coke bottle molds and remove bubbles on the poured mixture.
4. Place in the fridge for 1 to 2 hours before popping them out of the mold.

FRUITY ORANGE JELLY CANDY

Serves: 81

Nutritional Information (per serving):
Calories: 14 | Calories From Fat: 0 | Total Fat: 0 |
Total Carbohydrates: 3 g | Net Carbohydrates: 3 g | Protein: 0

INGREDIENTS:

- 2 tsp butter
- 3/4 oz powdered fruit pectin
- 1/2 tsp baking soda
- 3/4 cup water
- 1 cup sweetener, granulated
- 1 cup light corn syrup
- 1/8 tsp orange oil
- 5 drops red food color
- 5 drops yellow food color

DIRECTIONS:

1. Line a 9x9-inch pan with two tsp of butter.
2. Combine the pectin, baking soda, and water in a large saucepan. The mixture will look foamy. Bring to a boil.
3. In a separate saucepan, combine sweetener and corn syrup. Bring the mixture to a boil, around 4 minutes.
4. Slowly add in in the boiled pectin mixture on the sweetener mixture and boil for one minute while stirring constantly.
5. Remove from heat. Stir in the orange oil and food coloring.
6. Pour onto the 9-inch pan immediately and let it stand for 3 hours under room temperature.
7. Dip a knife in warm water and slice the firm jelly into 1-inch square sizes. Place on a rack and let it stand uncovered at room temperature overnight.

CREAMY ORANGE GUMMY

Serves: 4

Nutritional Information (per serving):
Calories: 119 | Calories From Fat: 99 | Total Fat: 11 g |
Total Carbohydrates: 1 g | Net Carbohydrates: 1 g | Protein: 2 g

INGREDIENTS:

- 0.3 oz Jell-O orange, sugar-free
- 2 envelopes unflavored gelatin
- 1 tbsp swerve powdered sweetener
- 1/2 cup cold water
- 1/2 cup heavy cream

DIRECTIONS:

1. In a small bowl, soften the unflavored gelatin in cold water.
2. Heat a small saucepan on medium heat and simmer the cream.
3. Add Jell-O and sweetener and mix until dissolved. Pour the softened gelatin and mix until dissolved.
4. Remove from heat and pour in candy silicone mold or pour in a loaf pan and cut after it sets.
5. Chill 1-2 hours before removing from mold.
6. Keep refrigerated before serving.

CUCUMBER LIME GUMMY

Serves: 4

Nutritional Information (per serving):
Calories: 10 | Calories From Fat: 0 | Total Fat: 0 |
Total Carbohydrates: 0 | Net Carbohydrates: 0 | Protein: 2 g

INGREDIENTS:

- 225 g cucumber
- 3 g mint tea leaves
- 1/2 lime juice
- 10 g gelatin powder
- A dash of stevia

DIRECTIONS:

1. In a blender, combine all the ingredients except gelatin.
2. Strain the mixture into a small pot. Turn on stove at medium heat and start to simmer the mixture.
3. Add in the gelatin powder slowly and stir until completely dissolved. Strain the gelatin mixture into a clean container.
4. Pour the mixture into your ice cube tray and refrigerate 2 hours.
5. Pop out from tray to serve.

VANILLA GUMDROPS

Serves: 7

Nutritional Information (per serving):
Calories: 30 | Calories From Fat: 0 | Total Fat: 0 |
Total Carbohydrates: 1 g | Net Carbohydrates: 0 | Protein: 5 g

INGREDIENTS:

- 5 cups filtered water
- 2 tbsp dried vanilla leaves
- 1/4 tsp citric acid
- 1 tbsp grated lemon zest
- 6 micro-scoops stevia extract
- 1 pinch ginger
- 6 tbsp beef gelatin, grass fed
- 1/2 cup water
- 2 tsp vanilla extract
- 4 drops yellow food coloring

DIRECTIONS:

1. Infuse the vanilla leaves in 5 cups of water by boiling it for 5 minutes. Cool before straining and transferring to another pan.
2. Place the strained vanilla water back on the stove to heat again.
3. Combine 1/2 cup water and gelatin and add to the vanilla water. Stir and let it boil until the gelatin dissolves. Remove from heat.
4. Add the sweetener, citric acid, lemon zest, and ginger. Mix well until it turns into a golden hue.

5. Divide the mixture into 2 and add vanilla flavor and yellow food color on the one half.
6. Pour the mixture in the silicone mold and put in the fridge for minimum of 2 hours. The longer it is in the fridge, the firmer your gummy will get. Remove the gumdrops from your mold before serving.

CREAMY CHOCOLATE GUMMY

Serves: 4

Nutritional Information (per serving):
Calories: 21 | Calories From Fat: 9 | Total Fat: 1 g |
Total Carbohydrates: 1 g | Net Carbohydrates: 1 g | Protein: 3 g

INGREDIENTS:

- 1/4 cup cold water
- 0.5 oz gelatin
- 1/4 cup boiling water
- 20-25 drops stevia liquid
- 1 tbsp cocoa powder
- 1 tbsp coconut cream, canned

DIRECTIONS:

1. Dissolve gelatin in boiling water until there are no more lumps.
2. Combine cold water, stevia, cocoa powder, and coconut cream. Stir until completely mixed. Combine both mixes.
3. Using a dropper, fill the gummy bear mold with the mixture.
4. Refrigerate for 20 minutes or until it hardens.

GRAPE FLAVORED GUMMY

Serves: 5

Nutritional Information (per serving):
Calories: 14 | Calories From Fat: 0 | Total Fat: 0 |
Total Carbohydrates: 0 | Net Carbohydrates: 0 | Protein: 3.5 g

INGREDIENTS:

- 25 g gelatin powder, unflavored
- 1/3 cup boiling water
- 1/2 cup cold water
- 12 drops sweet leaf, sweet drop grape flavor
- 6 drops purple food coloring

DIRECTIONS:

1. In a microwaveable container, place boiling water and add gelatin powder. Whisk then place in microwave for 30 seconds.
2. Remove from microwave and whisk again. Add the cold water and continue whisking to combine.
3. Add the grape drops and whisk. Taste if you wish to add more flavoring. Add the food color to get a dark brown color. Place in bottle molds and remove bubbles on the poured mixture.
4. Place in the fridge for 1 to 2 hours before popping them out of the mold.

CARROT JUICE GUMMY

Serves: 60

Nutritional Information (per serving):
Calories: 1 | Calories From Fat: 0 | Total Fat: 0 |
Total Carbohydrates: 2 g | Net Carbohydrates: 2 g | Protein: 0

INGREDIENTS:

- 4 tbsp unflavored gelatin
- 2/3 cup carrot juice
- 9 tsp swerve sweetener
- 4 tbsp monk fruit syrup
- Cooking spray

DIRECTIONS:

1. Prepare a 6x6-inch pan and lightly spray with cooking spray.
2. In a bowl, soften the gelatin in 4 tbsp of water for 5 minutes.
3. In a small pan over medium heat, mix carrot juice, sweetener, and monk fruit and stir until well combined.
4. Add in the softened gelatin and stir until it dissolves.
5. Remove from stove and pour on prepared pan.
6. Cool before refrigerating to set.
7. Cut into your desired shape and serve.

GRAPEFRUIT GUMMY

Serves: 60

Nutritional Information (per serving):
Calories: 1 | Calories From Fat: 0 | Total Fat: 0 |
Total Carbohydrates: 2 g | Net Carbohydrates: 2 g | Protein: 0

INGREDIENTS:

- 4 tbsp unflavored gelatin
- 2/3 cup pink grapefruit juice
- 9 tsp swerve sweetener
- 4 tbsp monk fruit syrup

DIRECTIONS:

1. Prepare a 6x6-inch pan and lightly spray with cooking spray.
2. In a bowl, soften the gelatin in 4 tbsp of water for 5 minutes.
3. In a small pan over medium heat, mix grapefruit juice, sweetener and monk fruit and stir until well combined.
4. Add in the softened gelatin and stir until it dissolves.
5. Remove from stove and pour into prepared pan.
6. Cool before refrigerating to set.
7. Cut into your desired shape and serve.

COFFEE GUMMIES

Serves: 30

Nutritional Information (per serving):
Calories: 15 | Calories From Fat: 9 | Total Fat: 1 g |
Total Carbohydrates: 0 | Net Carbohydrates: 0 | Protein: 2 g

INGREDIENTS:

- 1 cup freshly brewed coffee
- 1 tbsp grass fed butter
- 1 tbsp coconut oil
- 1 tbsp vanilla extract
- 5 tbsp unflavored gelatin powder
- 1 tbsp swerve sweetener

DIRECTIONS:

1. Combine all ingredients in a blender and mix until it turns frothy.
2. Pour into a candy mold and refrigerate for 2 hours until set.
3. Pop out of the mold and serve.

PINK MARGARITA ADULT GUMMIES

Serves: 24

Nutritional Information (per serving):
Calories: 50 | Calories From Fat: 0 | Total Fat: 0 |
Total Carbohydrates: 2.2 g | Net Carbohydrates: 1.8 g | Protein: 3.2 g

INGREDIENTS:

- 10 fresh or frozen strawberries, hulled
- 2 oz silver tequila
- 3 tbsp gelatin powder, unflavored
- 2 tbsp erythritol
- 1 1/2 oz fresh lime juice

DIRECTIONS:

1. Mix the strawberries and tequila in a blender until it turns smooth.
2. Pour the strawberry mixture in a saucepan over low heat. Add in the gelatin powder, sweetener, and lime. Whisk until powder dissolves or about 5 minutes.
3. Continue to whisk and heat for about 10 minutes or until it turns thin and smooth in consistency.
4. Pour into a container with spout before pouring over the gummy worm mold.
5. Refrigerate for about 15 minutes or until it sets. Pop from the mold and serve.

VALENTINE HEART GUMMIES

Serves: 30

Nutritional Information (per serving):
Calories: 40 | Calories From Fat: 28 | Total Fat: 3 g |
Total Carbohydrates: 1 g | Net Carbohydrates: 0.8 g | Protein: 2 g

INGREDIENTS:

- 6 tbsp gelatin powder, unflavored
- 3/4 cup + 1 tbsp water
- 2 cups fresh or frozen strawberries
- 1 cup heavy whipping cream
- 1/2 tsp vanilla extract
- 4 drops of liquid stevia

DIRECTIONS:

1. Divide the gelatin powder and the water and combine into two separate bowls. Let the gelatin bloom.
2. Place the strawberries in a blender and press blitz. When done, pour the blitzed strawberries on a muslin cloth to squeeze the juice out and strain the pith. This will make your gummy smooth.
3. Warm the cream in a saucepan over medium-low heat for one minute. Do not let it boil.
4. Add one of the bowl of bloomed gelatin then stir until it melts. Turn off the heat and add the vanilla and half of the sweetener.
5. In a separate saucepan, add half of the strawberry mixture and simmer for 30 seconds over medium-low heat. Add the second bowl of bloomed gelatin and stir until it melts.
6. Remove from heat then add the remaining half of the strawberry mix and the remaining sweetener. Stir until

thoroughly mixed. Remove any visible froth with a spoon.
7. Place the cream mixture and strawberry mixture into two separate containers with a spout.
8. To layer and mold, use a silicone heart mold. Fill half of each mold with the strawberry mixture then refrigerate for 30 minutes.
9. Take out from the fridge then fill the mold with the cream mixture to cover the set strawberry mixture. Chill for 2 hours.
10. Pop the gummy from the mold and store in the fridge until ready to serve.

CONCLUSION

I'd like to thank you and congratulate you for transiting my lines from start to finish.

I hope this book was able to help you to understand and learn more about sugar and its effect on your body.

The next step is to try out these recipes and indulge yourself. You are now armed with more information so you know what will work and not work for you.

I wish you the best of luck!

Made in the USA
Monee, IL
26 November 2022

18524595R00036